Book Of Medical Terminology Made

Very Simple For You

Olatundun Solomon

olatundunsolomon@gmail.com

Olatundun Solomon has Honor Code Certificate from the University of Texas System edx. The course is 4.01x: Take Your Medicine-The Impact of Drug Development.

A Certified Alison Graduate with distinction in the course: Diploma in Nursing and Patient Care.

He has Honor Code Certificate from Harvard University through edx in the course PH201x: Health and Society.

He is Certified Alison Graduate with distinction in the course: Diploma in Human Nutrition.

He also has Honor Code Certificate from edx Karolinska Institutet in the course KIBEHMEDx: Behavioral Medicine: A Key to Better Health.

Medical terminology is made simply for you. There are Latin words that are used. This can be translated to the English word. It can be a word, or two, three or more combined together. It can have prefix, infix and suffix. It can be monosyllabic, disyllabic or polysyllabic. e.g. cardiology is the combination of cardio + logy (heart + study of). This means, the study of the heart, its diseases, treatment and prevention of diseases. That is very simple to know and apply in the medical field of practice. Another example is the pericardium. This is the combination of the word peri + cardium (around + heart). This means the tissues around the heart. That is very simple.

Medical terminology is used in the medical field. It is made very simple for you, to be able to know, write and understand.

It can be applied by medical practitioners, medical students, health workers and the general public in order to make health practices easy to by achieved for a better outcome. This makes diseases to be understood by using medical terms. Therapy is then done immediately(stat). Also prevention of diseases is practised.

The public can easily relate to medical doctors concerning any issues. The medical practitioner can diagnose and the patient can easily understand and act right.

Medical students can use it in classes and in examinations. They can read textbooks and it can be simple for them, because the medical terminologies are easily understand while reading.

Pseudo means false: pseudocrisis is pseudo+crisis which is interpreted as false crisis.

Proto is early. For example,

protoplass is substance from which

cells are made.

Pleio is interpreted as excess. For

example, pleocytosis is interpreted

as many lymphocytes in the

cerebrospinal fluid (CSF) that is not

normal.

Plegia is interpreted as paralysis. For

example, hemiplegia (hemi + plegia)

is the combination of half+paralysis.

This is interpreted as paralysis that

occur to half part of the body.

Platy is interpreted as flat. For example, platyhelminth(platy+helminth) is the combination of flat+worm. This is interpreted as flat worm.

Plasty is interpreted as plastic surgery. For example, colonoplasty(colono+plasty) is the combination of colon+plastic surgery. This is interpreted as surgical reconstruction of a damaged colon(part of the large intestine).

Plasia is interpreted as formation.

For example, hyperplasia(

hyper+plasia) is (excess+formation).

This is interpreted as excess tissue

formation.

Pimelo is interpreted as fat. For

example, pimelotomy(pimelo+tomy)

is (fat+surgical incision) is

interpreted as the surgical incision

that is made, in order to remove fat.

Pilo is interpreted as hair. For

example, pilomotor nerves is

interpreted as muscle tissues around

the hair, supplied by sympathetic

nerve root.

Phyto this is interpreted as plants.

For example,

phytotherapy(phyto+therapy) is

interpreted as (plant+treatment).

This is the treatment that occur by

using plant.

Physio is interpreted as physical. For

example, physiotherapy

(physio+therapy) is

(physical+healing). This is the

physical method that is used for

healing to occur.

Physo is interpreted as air. For

example,

physopharmacotherapy(physo+phar

maco+therapy). This is

(air+drug+healing). This is the use of

inhaler (air+drug) as method for

healing.

Phren is interpreted as the

diaphragm. For example, phrenic

nerve is the nerve that innervates

the diaphragm.

Phrenia is interpreted as the condition of the mind. For example, schizophrenia(schizo+phrenia) which is (division+mind). This is illness of the mind that is severe.

Phon is interpreted as sound. For example, phonation is the production of vocal sound.

Phobia is interpreted as fear. For example, agoraphobia(agora+phobia) is (open place+fear). Which is fear of public places.

Photo is interpreted as light. For example, photodermatosis(photo+dermatosis), is (light+skin diseases). Which is disease of the skin from light.

Phoria is interpreted as deviation that is not normal that is of the eye. For example, heterophoria(hetero+phoria). This is (other+deviation that is not normal). Which is deviation of the other eye when one is closed.

Phlebo is interpreted as vein. For example, phlebothrombosis is (phlebo+thrombosis). This is (vein+blood clot that cause blockage). Which is when the vein experience blockage as a result of blood clot.

Philia is interpreted as attraction. For example, philia is (pharmaco+philia). This is (drug+attraction). Which is attraction to drug. This may happen after somebody is sick. After taken drug for that sickness such person can then be healed.

Phanero is interpreted as visible. For example, phanerorrhoea is(phanero+rrhoea). This is (visible+flow), which is visible flow of liquid.

Pharmaco is interpreted as drugs. For example, pharmacotherapy is (pharmaco+therapy). This is (drugs+treatment), which is the use of drugs for the treatment of diseases.

Pexy is interpreted as fixation that occurred surgically. For example, jejunopexy is (jejuno+pexy). This is (jejunum+fixation). Which is fixation of the jejunum.

Phaco is interpreted as eye lens. For example, phacopathy is (phaco+pathy). This is (lens+ disease), which is disease of the lens of the eyes.

Phagia is interpreted as eating. For example, bacteriophagia is (bacterio+phagia). Is (bacteria+eating), which is bacteria is eating up, or destroyed by white blood cells.

Pero is interpreted as defect. For example, perocardial. This is (pero+cardial) is (defect+heart). Which is heart defect.

Peri is interpreted as around. For example, pericardium is (peri+cardium). Is (around+heart). Which is tissues around the heart.

Pericardio is interpreted as pericardium. For example,

pericardiocele is (pericardio+cele) is (pericardium + swelling). Which is swelling of the pericardium.

Pent is interpreted as five. For example, pentose is(pent+ose). This is (five+sugar). Which is five carbon atom sugar.

Para is interpreted as close. For example parasternal is(para+sternal). This is (close+sternum). Which is close to the sternum.

Papulo is interpreted as pimples. For example papulotherapy is (papulo+therapy). This is (pimples+treatment). Which is treatment of the pimples.

Pan is interpreted as general. For example, pananaesthesia is (pan+anaesthesia). This is (general+loss of sensation). Which is general body loss of sensation. This can be achieved by the administration of general

anaesthetic.

Pali this is interpreted as repetition.

For example, palipathy is

(pali+pathy). This is

(repetition+disease). Which is

repetition of disease.

Palato is interpreted as the palate.

For example, palatoplasty is

(palato+plasty). This is

(palate+plastic surgery). Which is

plastic surgery of the palate.

Palaeo is interpreted as primitive. For example, palaeomelia is (palaeo+melia). This is (primitive+limbs). Which is primitive limbs of the foetus in the uterus of a pregnant woman.

Paed is interpreted as children. For example, paediatrics is (paed+iatrics). This is (children+medicine). Which is children general medicine specialty.

Ovi is interpreted as ovum. For example, oviduct is (ovi+duct). This is (ovum+tube). Which is fallopian tube through which ovum passes after fertilization and is implanted in the uterus.

Ovari is interpreted as ovary. For example ovarian cyst is the tumour of the ovary.

Osmo is interpreted as osmosis. For example, osmoreceptor is (osmo+receptor). This is (osmosis+receptor). Which is receptors of cells in the hypothalamus that helps in osmosis to monitor blood concentration.

Osis is interpreted as disease condition. For example, leucocytosis is (leukocyt+osis). This is (white blood cell+disease condition). Which is increase in white blood cells in a disease condition.

Osche is interpreted as the scrotum. For example, oscheitis is (osche+itis). This is (scrotum+inflammation). Which is inflammation of the scrotum.

Ortho is interpreted as normal. For example, orthophoria is

(ortho+phoria). This is (normal +condition of the eye alignment). Which is normal alignment condition of the eyes.

Organo is interpreted as organ. Organopathy is (organo+pathy). This is (organ+disease). Which is disease of an organ in the body.

Sapr is interpreted as decaying matter caused by saprophytic bacteria. For example, sapraemia is (sapr+aemia). This is (decaying matter in the blood as poison. This is caused by saprophytic bacteria.

Sanguino is interpreted as blood. For example sanguinorrhge, is (sanguino+rrhage). This is (blood+excess flow). Which is blood excess flow from damaged vessel.

Salping is interpreted as fallopian tube. For example salpingitis is (salping+itis). This is (fallopian tube+inflammation). Which is fallopian tube inflammation.

Sacro this is interpreted as sacrum.
For example sacroiliac joint. Is the
joint between the sacrum and the
ilium.

Rhizo is interpreted as root. For
example, rhizotomy is (rhizo+tomy).
This is (root+cut by making incision).
Which is when nerve roots are cut
from the spinal cord.

Rheo is interpreted as when there is
flow of liquid. For example,
rheohidrosis(rheo+hidrosis). This is
(flow of liquid+sweat excretion).

Which is the excretion of sweat and the liquid flows.

Retin is interpreted as retina. For example, retinitis is (retin+itis). This is (retina+inflammation). Which is retina inflammation.

Recto is interpreted as rectum. For example, rectocele is (recto+cele). This is (rectum+pouching). Which is pouching that occur to the rectum.

Quadri is interpreted as four. For example, quadriplegia is (quadri+plegia). This is (four+paralysis). Which is the four limbs paralysis.

Pylor is interpreted as pylorus. For example, pyloric stenosis is the narrowing of the stomach outlet pylorus.

Pyle is interpreted as portal vein. For example, pylethrombosis is (pyle+thrombosis). This is (portal vein + obstruction of blood vessel by blood clot). Which is portal vein obstruction by blood clot.

Pygo is interpreted as buttocks. For example, pygopathy is (pygo+pathy). This is disease of the buttocks.

Pykno is interpreted as thickness. For example, pyknosis is when the cell nucleus becomes thickened.

Pyelo is interpreted as pelvis of the kidney. For example, pyelocystitis is (pyelo+cyst+itis). This is (pelvis of the kidney+urinary bladder+inflammation). Which is pelvis of the kidney and urinary bladder inflammation.

Py is interpreted as pus. For example, pyarthrosis is (py+arthrosis). This is (pus+disease condition of the joint). Which is pus in the disease condition of the joint.

Pulmo is interpreted as lungs. For example, pulmonary embolism is embolus obstructing the pulmonary artery.

Pterygo is interpreted as sphenoid bone pterygoid process.

Psych is interpreted as the mind. For example, psychiatry is (psych+iatry).

This is (mind+study). Which is the study of the mind (mental) disorder. And also how it can be prevented and managed in a medical specialty.

Splanch is interpreted as viscera. For example, Splanchnic nerves innervates the viscera.

Spino is interpreted as spinal cord. For example, spinocerebellar degeneration is cerebellum and also the corticospinal tract disorder.

Sphygmo is interpreted as pulse. For example, sphygmoscope is (sphygmo+scope). That is (pulse+to instrument for observing). Which is instrument that is used for observing pulse.

Sphinctero is sphincter. For example, sphincterotomy is (sphinctero+tomy). This is (sphincter+in incision made to remove). Which is surgical incision made, in order to remove the sphincter.

Spermio is interpreted as sperm. For example, spermiogenesis is (spermio+genesis). This is (sperm+development). Which is development of spermatid into spermatozoa.

Spermato is interpreted as sperm. For example, spermatocyte is (spermato+cyte). This is (sperm+cell). Which is in between stage of sperm cell of spermatozoa.

Spasmo is interpreted as spasm. For example, spasmolytic is drug that is used for relieving smooth muscle spasm.

Somat is interpreted as body. For example, somatopleure is early embryo body wall.

skia is interpreted as shadow. For example skiaphobia is (skia+phobia). That is (shadow+fear), which is fear of shadow.

Sigmoid is interpreted as sigmoid colon. For example sigmoidoscopy is the use of instrument to examine the sigmoid colon and the rectum.

Sialo is interpreted as saliva. For example, sialorrhoea is when saliva is produced in excess.

Sero is interpreted as serum. For example, serofibrinous is (sero+fibrinous). This is many protein fibrin in serum.

Septi is interpreted as sepsis. For example, septicaemia is bacteria that can cause disease are in the blood. And this cause destruction of tissues.

Sclero is interpreted as thickening.

For example, scleroderma is

(sclero+derma). This is

(thickening+skin), which when the

skin is thickened.

Schizo is interpreted as division. For

example, schizophrenia is mental

(mind) disorder.

Vulv is interpreted as vulva. For

example, vulvectomy is

(vulv+ectomy). That is

(vulva+excision to remove). Which is

surgical removal of the vulva.

Video is recording and observation

of images are done by video camera.

For example, video-otoscope is used

to examine the ear.

Vesico is interpreted as urinary

bladder. For example, vesicostomy is

(vesico+stomy). This is (urinary

bladder+opening or channel). Which

is surgical making of an opening or

channel for the flow of urine liquid,

between the bladder and the skin.

Tetano is interpreted as tetanus. For

example, tetanospasmin is muscle

spasm caused by poison from

tetanus bacilli.

Thalam is interpreted as thalamus.

For example, thalamic syndrome

occurred as a result of thalamus

trauma.

Teno is interpreted as tendon. For

example, tenoplasty is

(tendon+plastic surgery). Which is

plastic surgery done, in order to

repair ruptured tendon.

Terato is interpreted as congenital

abnormality. For example,

teratogenesis is (terato+genesis). This is (congenital abnormality+ origin of development). Which is occurrence resulting to developmental abnormality to the foetus in the uterus.

Temporo is interpreted as the temporal bone. For example, temporomandibular joint. Is the joint between the temporal bone and the mandible bone.

Tele is interpreted as distance. For example, teleceptor is (tele+ceptor).

This is (distance+receptor). Which is receptor that can respond to stimuli that is at distance.

Tars is interpreted as the tarsal bones. For example, tarsalgia is (tars+algia). This is (tarsal bones+pain). Which is pain in the tarsal bones.

Talo is interpreted as talus. For example, talotibial joint is is the joint between the talus and the tibia.

Syndesm is interpreted as connective tissue. For example,

syndesmosis is connective tissue

separating immovable joint.

Stylo is interpreted as the styloid

process of the temporal bone. For

example, stylohyoid muscle. This is

from the styloid process of the

temporal bone to the bone of the

hyoid.

Sub is interpreted as below. For

example, subdural is (sub+dural).

This is (below+dura). Which is below

the dura matter.

Stomy is interpreted as opening surgically. For example, duodenostomy is surgical opening into the duodenum.

Sterno is interpreted as sternum. For example, sternocostal is (sterno+costal). This is (sternum+rib). Which is the sternum and the rib.

Squamo is interpreted as squamous epithelium. For example squamous cell carcinoma is cancer of the squamous epithelium.

Spondylo is interpreted as the vertebra. For example, spondylolysis. This is when the vertebra as bony defect.

Splen is interpreted as spleen. For example splenitis is (splen+itis). This is (spleen+inflammation). Which is inflammation of the spleen.

Arterio is interpreted as artery. For example, arteriography is(arterio+graphy). This is (artery+diagram or image). Which is image of the artery that is done by

an instrument.

Archi is interpreted as primitive. For

example, archicardia is

(archi+cardiac). This is

(primitive+heart). Which is primitive

embryonic heart that is formed in

the uterus of a pregnant woman.

Ante is interpreted as before. For

example, anterior is the front part of

the body.

Anti is interpreted as counteracting.

For example, antiseptic. This is

(anti+septic). This is (against or

counteracting+disease causing

microorganisms). Which is, is against

or destroy disease causing

microorganisms.

Anglo is interpreted as blood vessel.

For example, angiogenesis is

(Anglo+genesis). This is (blood

vessel+new formation or origin).

Which is formation of new blood

vessel.

Algia is interpreted as pain. For

example, abdominalgia is

(abdomin+algia). This is (

abdomen+pain). Which is pain in the

abdomen of the body.

Andro is interpreted as men. For

example, androgenization. This the

occurrence of male sexual

characteristics, as a result of the

hormone androgen.

Adeno is interpreted as gland. For

example, adenocarcinoma. This is

(adeno+carcinoma). This is

(gland+cancer). Which is cancer

tumour formation in a gland.

Ad is interpreted as towards. For example, adnasal is (ad+nasal). This is (towards+nose). Which is towards the nose.

Acro is interpreted as extremity. For example, acrodermatitis is (acro +dermat+itis). This is (extremity+skin+inflammation). Which is extremity of the body hands and feet the skin, as inflammation.

A is interpreted as absence of. For example, atoxic is (a+toxic). This is (absence of+toxin or poison). Which is absence of poison.

Ab is interpreted as away. For example, abduct is the movement away from the midline by a limb.

Abdomin is interpreted as abdomen. For example, abdominitis is (abdomin+itis). This is (abdomen+inflammation). Which is when inflammation occur to the abdomen.

Xiphi is interpreted as the sternum xiphoid process. For example, xiphisternal joint. Is the joint between the xiphoid process of the sternum and the sternum body.

Xero is interpreted as when a condition is dry. For example, xerosis is the abnormal dryness of mucous membrane of the skin.

Xeno is interpreted as foreign. For example, xenodiagnosis is foreign body such as microorganisms diagnosis.

Xantho is interpreted as yellow colour. For example, xanthoma is yellow skin that is having lesion.

Cac is interpreted as disease. For example, cacencephalon is (cac+encephalon). This is (disease+brain). Which is disease of the brain.

Broncho is interpreted as bronchial tree. For example, bronchodilator is (broncho+dilator). This is (bronchial tree+drug that dilate). Which is drug that dilate the bronchial tree.

Brady is interpreted as slowness. For example, bradycardia is (brady+cardia). This is (slowness+heart). Which is slowness of the heart rate.

Brachi is interpreted as arm. For example, brachialis is muscle formed at the arm.

Brachy is interpreted as shortness. For example, brachybrachial is (shortness+arm). Which is shortness of the arm.

Blephero is interpreted as eyelid. For example, blepharospasm is tight contraction of the eyelid.

Blenno is interpreted as mucus. For example, blennorrhoea is (blenno+rrhoea). This is (mucus+discharge). Which is discharge of mucus.

Blast is interpreted as formative cell. For example, neuroblast is (neuron+formative cell). Which is neuron formative cell.

Blasto is interpreted as embryo. For example, blastocoele is (blasto+coele). This is (embryo+fluid filled). Which is embryo that as fluid filled cavity in blastocyst.

Bio is interpreted as life. For example, biopsy is when living tissue is removed.removed

Bili is interpreted as bile. For example, bilious is having bile.

Bi is interpreted as two. For example, biceps muscle of the body that has two heads.

Azo is interpreted as urea. For example, azoturia is urea in the urine.

Auxo is interpreted as growth. For example, auxocranium is growth of the cranium.

Auto is interpreted as self or involuntarily. For example, autonomic nervous system. This nervous system occurs involuntarily in the body.

Audio means hearing. For example audiometer is (audio+meter). This is

(audio+instrument that measure).

Which is instrument that measure

for testing of hearing.

Atrio is interpreted as atrium. For

example, the atrioventricular

septum is septum between the

atrium and the ventricle.

Ase is interpreted as enzyme. For

example, amylase. This is enzyme

that digest amylose.

Arthur is interpreted as joint. For

example, arthrectomy is

(arthr+ectomy). This is

(joint+excision). Which is joint excision.

Chord is interpreted as notochord. For example, chordoma is (chord+oma). This is (notochord+tumour). Which is notochord remnant tumour of the embryo.

Chondro is interpreted as cartilage. For example, chondroclast is cell that absorbs cartilage.

Choledocho is interpreted as common bile duct. For example,

choledocholithiasis is common bile

duct that is having stone.

Chol is interpreted as bile. For

example, cholagogue is drug that

cause bile flow.

Cholecyst is interpreted as gall

bladder. For example,

cholecystectomy is

(cholecyst+ectomy). This is (gall

bladder+excision). Which is gall

bladder removal by making excision.

Chlor is interpreted as green. For

example, chloropsia is green vision.

Chir is interpreted as hand. For example, chiralgia is (chir+algia). This is (hand+pain). Which is hand pain.

Cheil is interpreted as lips. For example, cheilosis, is swollen lips.

Cervic is interpreted as the cervix. For example, cervicitis is (cervix+inflammation). Which is inflammation of the cervix.

Cerebro is interpreted as cerebrum. For example, cerebrospinal fluid. Is fluid that flows in the cerebrum and

in the spinal cord.

Central is interpreted as centre. For

example, centripetal is going

towards the centre.

Centesis is interpreted as

perforation. For example,

chordocentesis is perforation of

umbilical vein by using fine needle in

order to remove fetal blood. This can

be used for blood test.

Coele is interpreted as swelling. For example, hepatocoele is swelling of the liver.

Cata is interpreted as downward or degenerated. For example, cataplasia is tissue degeneration.

Carp is interpreted as carpus(wrist). For example, carpometacarpal joint is the joint between the carpus and metacarpus.

Cardiac is interpreted as heart. For example, carditis is the inflammation of the heart.

Carcin is interpreted as cancer. For example, carcinogen is something can can cause cancer.

Calc is interpreted as calcium. For example, calculi is calcium salt stone. This can be found in the kidney known as kidney stone.

Cyto is interpreted as cell. For example, cytopathy is (cyto+pathy). This is (cell+disease). Which is cell disease.

Cyte is interpreted as cell. For example, erythrocytes is

(erythro+cytes). This is (red+cells).

Which is red blood cells.

Cysto is the urinary bladder. For

example, cystotomy is (cysto+tomy).

This is (urinary bladder+incision).

Which is urinary bladder incision.

Cyclo is interpreted as the ciliary

body. For example, cyclopathy is

(cyclo+pathy). This is (ciliary body

+disease). Which is disease of the

ciliary body.

Cryo is interpreted as cold. For

example, cryosurgery is using cold

(very low temperature) to destroy

unwanted tissue by freezing part of

the human body.

Cranio is interpreted as the skull. For

example, craniopagus is conjoined

heads of twins.

Coxo is interpreted as the hip. For

example, coxoplegia is (coxo+plegia).

This is (hip+paralysis). Which is the

hip paralysis.

Cost is interpreted as the ribs. For

example, costal is associated with

the ribs.

Copro is interpreted as faeces. For example, coprolith is (copro+lith). This is (faeces+hardened). Which is hardened faeces.

Contra is interpreted as opposite. For example, contralateral is when opposite part of the body is affected.

Colp is interpreted as the vagina. For example, colpitis is (colp+itis). This is (vagina+inflammation). Which is inflammation of the vagina.

Colono is interpreted as colon. For example, colonorraphy is (colono+rraphy). This is

(colon+surgical suturing). Which is

tear of the colon that surgically

suturing it is used as treatment.

Coeli is interpreted as abdomen. For

example, coelipathy is (coeli+pathy).

This (abdomen+disease). Which is

disease of the abdomen.

Cleido is interpreted as the clavicle.

For example, sternocleidomastoid

muscle is attached to the sternum,

clavicle and the mastoid bone.

Coccy is interpreted as the coccyx.

For example, coccyalgia is

(coccy+algia). This is (coccyx+pain).

Which is pain from the coccyx.

Cirs is interpreted as varicose vein.

For example, cirsoid is appearance of

varicose vein.

Cine is interpreted as cinefilm. X-ray

images are recorded by it. For

example, cineangiography the

imaging of blood vessels by using

cine film to record it.

Cide is interpreted as killing. For example, pesticide is (pesti+cide). This is (pest+killing). Which is pest killing chemical.

Chrys is gold. For example, chrysiasis is gold present in tissue.

Chrono is interpreted as time. For example, chronophilia is (chrono+philia). This is (time+attraction). Which is attraction to time by looking at the clock.

Chromato is interpreted as pigmentation. For example, chromatophore is pigmentation of cell.

Ectro is interpreted as absence. For example, ectrodactyly is (ectro+dactyly). This is (absence+fingers). Which is when there is absence of the fingers congenitally.

Ectomy is interpreted as removal. For example, colonectomy is (colon+ectomy). This is (colon+removal), which is removal of the colon surgically.

Ecto is interpreted as outer. For example, ectoderm is the outer germ layer.

Ec is interpreted as outside. For example, ecdemic is disease from outside country.

Dynia is interpreted as pain. For example, abdominodynia is (abdomino+dynia). This is (abdomen+pain). Which is pain in the abdomen.

Dys is interpreted as abnormal. For example, dyscoria is when the pupil is having abnormal shape.

Duo is interpreted as two. For example, duobrachium is (duo+brachium). This is (two+arm). Which is two arms.

Dor is interpreted as back. For example, dorsal is back part of the body.

Duoden is interpreted as duodenum. For example, duodenitis is (duoden+itis). This is (duodenum+inflammation). Which is

inflammation of the duodenum.

Dolicho is interpreted as long. For

example, dolichobrachium is

(dolicho+brachium). This is

(long+arm). Which is long arm.

Dis is interpreted as separation. For

example, disarticulation is

separation of joint.

Dia is interpreted as through. For

example, diarrhoea is (dia+rrhoea).

This is (through+flow). Which is

frequent discharge of soft and

watery wastes due to infection, that flow through the intestines and come out through the anus.

Di is interpreted as two. For example, disarccharide. This two monosaccharide.

Dextro is interpreted as right side. For example, dextrobrachium is (dextro+brachium). This is (right side +arm). Which is the arm at the right side.

Deuto is interpreted as two. For example, deutobrachia is

(deuto+brachia). This is (two+arms).

Which is two arms.

Derm is interpreted as germ layer.

For example, endoderm is (

endo+derm). This is (inner+germ

layer). Which is inner germ layer.

Dermato is interpreted as skin. For

example, dermatosis is disease

condition of the skin.

Dent is interpreted as teeth. For

example, dental care. This is care of

the teeth.

Demi is is interpreted as half. For example, demiplegia is (demi+plegia). This is (half+paralysis). Which is paralysis of half part of the body.

Deci is interpreted as tenth. For example, decibel is (deci+bel). This is (tenth+bel). Which is a tenth of bel.

De is interpreted as loss. For example, dehydrate is loss of water from the body.

Dactyl is interpreted as fingers or toes. For example, dactylalgia is (dactyl+algia). This is (fingers or toes

+ pain). Which is pain in the fingers

or toes.

Gastr is interpreted as stomach. For

example, gastritis is (gastr+itis). This

is (stomach+inflammation). Which is

inflammation of the stomach.

Fuge is interpreted as agent that

eliminates. For example,

bacteriofuge is (bacterio+fuge). This

is (bacteria+agent that eliminates).

Which is agent that eliminates

bacteria.

Flavo is interpreted as yellow. For example, flavoderm is (flavor+derm). This is (yellow+skin). Which is when the skin is yellow in appearance.

Fibro is interpreted as fibres. For example, fibrocartilaginous. This is combination of fibres and cartilage.

Feto is interpreted as fetus. For example, fetoscopy is an instrument (endoscopy) that is used to view the fetus.

Ferri is interpreted as iron. For example, ferritin is known as iron protein complex.

Facio is interpreted as face. For example, facioplegia is (facio+plegia). This is (face+paralysis). Which is paralysis of the face.

Facient is interpreted as causing. For example, auxofacient is (auxo+facient). This is (growth+causing). Which is causing growth.

Extra is interpreted as outside. For example, extracellular is (extra+cellular). This is happening outside cell.

Ex is interpreted as outer. For example, excrescence is outward growth that is abnormal.

Eu is interpreted as normal. For example, eucardia is normal heart.

Erythro is interpreted as redness. For example, erythrocyte is red blood cell.

Ergo is interpreted as activity. For example, ergocardia is activity of the heart.

Episio is interpreted as vulva. For example, episiorrhaphy is (episio+rraphy). This is (vulva+surgical suturing). Which is surgical suturing of the vulva.

Epiplo is interpreted as momentum. For example, epiplopathy is (epiplo+pathy).This is (omentum+disease). Which is disease of the omentum.

Epi is interpreted as above. For example, epicondyle is (epi+condyle). This is (above+condyle). Which is a protuberance that is above the condyle.

Enter is interpreted as intestine. For example, enteritis is (enter+itis). This is (intestine+inflammation). Which is inflammation of the intestine.

Endo is interpreted as inner. For example, endoderm is (endo+derm). This is (inner+germ layer). Which is inner layer of the germ layer.

En is interpreted as inside. For

example, encephalon is

(en+cephalon). This is (inside+head).

Which is the brain inside the head.

Gynaeco is interpreted as is female.

For example, gynaecology is

(gynaeco+logy). This is

(female+study of). Which is the

study of the female disease.

Gonio is interpreted as angle. For

example, gonion is angle of the

mandible.

Glyco is interpreted as sugar. For example, glycogen is glucose sugar that is stored in the liver.

Gluco is interpreted as glucose. Glucose is six carbon sugar.

Glosso is interpreted as tongue. For example, glossopathy is (glosso+pathy). This is (tongue+disease). Which is disease of the tongue.

Gli is interpreted as glia. For example, glioma is (gli+oma). This is (glia+tumour). Which is tumour of glia.

Gingiv is interpreted as gums. For example, gingivitis is (gingiv+itis). This is (gums+inflammation). Which is inflammation of the gums.

Ger is interpreted old age. For example, geriatric. This is diagnosis and treatment of old age people.

Genic is interpreted as producing. For example, erythrocytogenic is producing of red blood cells.

Genesis is interpreted as as development. For example, splenogenesis is (spleno+genesis). This is (spleen+development). Which is development of the spleen.

Genito is interpreted as organs of reproduction. For example, genitopathy is (genito+pathy). This is (reproduction organs+disease). Which is disease of organs of reproduction.

Orchio is interpreted as testicle. For example, orchiopathy is (orchio+pathy). This is

(testicle+disease). Which is disease

of the testicle.

Opt is interpreted as eye. For

example, opticokinetic is eye

movement.

Opia is interpreted as eye defect. For

example, myopia is short

sightedness.

Oophoro is interpreted as ovary. For

example, oophoropexy is

(oophoro+pexy). This is

(ovary+surgical fixation). Which is

surgical fixation of ovary that as been displaced.

Ophthalm is interpreted as eye. Ophthalmia is inflammation of the eye.

Oo is interpreted as ovum. For example, oocyte is cell in the ovary through meiosis forms ovum.

Oneiro is interpreted as dream. For example, oneironormocardial is (oneiro+normo+cardinal). This is (dream+normal+heart). Which is dream that is the heart is in normal condition.

Onycho is interpreted as nail. For example, Onychomycosis is nails infected by fungus.

Omphalo is interpreted as umbilical cord. For example, omphalocele is (omphalo+cele). This is (umbilical cord +hernia). Which is hernia of the umbilicus.

Oesophago is interpreted as oesophagus. For example, oesophagotomy is (oesophago+tomy). This is

(oesophagus+incision made to open).

Which is making incision surgically,

to open the oesophagus.

Nympho is interpreted as labia

minora. For example, nymphorraphy

is (nympho+rrhaphy). This is (labia

minors +surgical suture repair).

Which is surgical suture repair of the

labia minors that as torn.

Nycto is interpreted as darkness. For

example, nyctophobia is

(nycto+phobia). This is

(darkness+fear). Which is the fear of darkness.

Noct is interpreted as night. For example, noctodontodynia is (nocto+donto+dynia). This is (night+teeth+pain). Which is teeth pain at night.

Noci is interpreted as pain. For example, nociceptor is sensation of pain receptor.

Neo is interpreted as new. For example, neonatal teeth is teeth of the first month of life.

Naso is interpreted as nose. For example, nasolacrimal is the lacrimal apparatus and the nose.

Narco is interpreted as unconsciousness. For example, narcotic is drug that cause unconsciousness.

Oculo is interpreted as eye. For example, oculopathy is (oculo+pathy). This is (eye+disease). Which is eye disease.

Eu is interpreted as normal. For example, eucardium is (eu+cardium).

This is (normal+heart). Which is normal heart.

Ventricul is interpreted as the ventricle of the heart or brain. For example, ventriculitis is (ventricul+itis). This is (ventricle+inflammation). Which is inflammation of the ventricle.

Vene is interpreted as the vein. For example, venepuncture is (vene+puncture). This is (vein+puncture). Which is vein puncture that is done in order to

remove blood for blood test.

Vaso is interpreted as vessel. For

example, vasoconstriction is

(vaso+constriction). Which is

constriction of blood vessel.

Urin is interpreted as urine. For

example, urinary bladder. Is bladder

that urine is stored into.

Tricho is interpreted as hair.

Trichopathy is (tricho+pathy). This is

(hair+disease). Which is disease of

the hair.

Pilo is interpreted as hair. For example, pilopathy is (pilo+pathy). This is (hair+disease). Which is disease of the hair.

Uria is interpreted as condition of the urine. For example, polyuria is when urine is produced in large volume.

Tono is interpreted as pressure. For example, tonometer is (tono+meter). This is (pressure+instrument that is used for measuring). Which is instrument that is used for measuring the pressure inside the eye.

Urethro is interpreted as urethra. For example, urethrocele is (urethro+cele). This is (urethra+tumour). Which is tumour of the urethra.

Tachy is interpreted as fast. For example, tachycardia is (tachy+cardia). This is (fast+heart). Which is fast heart rate.

Tibio is interpreted as tibia. For example, tibiotalal joint is the joint between the tibia and the talus bone.

Thymia is interpreted as the condition of the mind. For example, euthymia is (eu+thymia). This is (normal+condition of the mind). Which is normal condition of the mind.

Supra is interpreted as above. For example, suprarenal glands. These are glands above the kidneys.

Sub is interpreted as below. For example, subclavius is below the clavicle.

Uran is the palate. For example, uranitis is (uran+itis). Which is the inflammation of the palate.

Stomato is interpreted as the mouth. For example, stomatopathy is (stomato+pathy). This is (mouth+disease). Which is disease of the mouth.

Stetho is interpreted as chest. For example, stethoscope is an instrument that is used to auscultate the chest.

Sterco is interpreted as faeces. For example, stercolith is (sterco+lith). This is (faeces+hard). Which is hard faeces.

Stasis is interpreted as stoppage. For example, haemostasis is (haemo+stasis). This is (blood+stoppage). Which is stoppage of blood flow.

Steato is interpreted as fatty tissue.

For example, steatotomy is fatty

tissue removal.

Steno is interpreted as narrow. For

example, stenosis is narrow blood

vessel.

Spiro is interpreted as respiration.

For example, spirometer is

(spiro+meter). This is

(respiration+measuring instrument).

Which is instrument used in

measuring inspiration and expiration

during respiration.

Sito is interpreted as food. For

example, sitosepsis is food infection.

Sinistro is interpreted as left. For

example, sinistrobrachium is

(sinistro+brachium). This is

(left+arm). Which is left arm.

Sarc is interpreted as muscle. For

example, sarcoma is (sarc+oma).

This is (muscle+tumour). Which is

tumour of the muscle.

Rrhagia is interpreted as excessive

flow from part of the body. For

example, haemorrhagia is

(haemo+rrhagia). This is

(blood+excessive flow from part of

the body). Which is blood excessive

flow from part of the body that is

traumatized.

Rhino is interpreted as nose. For

example, otorhinolaryngology is

(oto+rhino+laryngo+logy). This is

(ear+nose+throat+study of). Which

is the study of the ear, nose and

throat.

Tropho is interpreted as nutrition.

For example, trophocardia is

(tropho+cardiac). This is

(nutrition+heart). Which is nutrition

of the heart.

Reno is interpreted as kidney. For

example, renolith is (reno+lith). This

is (kidney+stone). Which is kidney

stone.

Tomo is interpreted as surgical

operation. For example, tomocardia

is surgical operation of the heart.

Pyr is interpreted as fever. Pyrexia is

fever.

Pyreto is interpreted as fever. For example, pyretosommatic is causes fever of the body.

Ptyalo is interpreted as siliva. For example, ptyalorrhoea is when siliva flow is too much.

Poiesis is interpreted as production. For example, erythropoiesis is red blood cell production.

Tracheo is interpreted as the trachea. For example, tracheotomy is (tracheo+tomy). This is (trachea+surgical incision to open).

Which is surgical incision made to the trachea to open it.

Pnoea is interpreted as breathing. For example, tachypnoea is (tachy+pnoea). This is (fast+breathing). Which is fast breathing.

Oto is interpreted as ear. For example, otorhinolaryngology is(oto+rhino+laryngo+logy). This is (ear+nose+throat+study of). Which is the study of the ear, nose and throat.

Osteo is interpreted as bone. For example, osteocyte is (osteo+cyte). This is (bone+cell). Which is bone cell.

Pod is interpreted as foot. For example, podiatry is the study of the foot. And also the care of it.

Opt is interpreted as eye. For example, optic nerve is nerve of the eye.

Onco is interpreted as tumour. For example, oncology is (onco+logy). This is (tumour+study of). Which is the study of tumour.

Omo is interpreted as shoulder. For example, omohyoid muscle is from the shoulder to the hyoid bone.

Oligo is interpreted as deficiency. For example, oligodontia is absence of some teeth congenitally.

Oma is interpreted as tumour. For example, lymphoma is tumour of the lymph nodes.

Pleuro is interpreted as pleura. For example, pleurocele is (pleuro+cele). This is (pleura+hernia). Which is hernia of the pleura.

Somn is interpreted as sleep. For example, insomnia is not able to sleep.

Tubo is interpreted as fallopian tube. For example, tubo-ovary is occurring in a fallopian tube and an ovary.

Odonto is interpreted as teeth. For example, odontology is (odonto+logy). This is (teeth+study of). Which is the study of the teeth.

Tome is interpreted as instrument that cut. For example, microtome is instrument that cut thin slice of

tissue.

Normo is interpreted as normal. For

example, normotension is normal

arterial blood pressure.

Noso is interpreted as disease. For

example, nosocephalon is

(noso+cephalon). This is

(disease+brain). Which is disease of

the brain.

Nephro is interpreted as kidney. For

example, nephron is the functional

part of the kidney. Filtration of blood occur in it.

Necro is interpreted as death. For example, necrospermia is spermatozoa that is dead.

Naso is interpreted as nose. For example, nasorraphy is (naso+rraphy). This (nose+surgical repair by suturing). Which is surgical repair of the nose that as torn, by suturing it.

Myxo is interpreted as mucus. For example, myxoedema is oedema that is having mucus in it.

Myo is interpreted as muscle. For example, myocytes is (myo+cytes). This is (muscle+cells). Which is muscle cells.

Musculo is interpreted as muscle. For example, musculoskeletal system. Is the system of the muscle and skeleton.

Muco is interpreted as mucus. For example, mucous membrane is membrane that produce mucus.

Mono is interpreted as one. For example, monosaccharide is (mono+saccharide). This is (one+sugar). Which is one sugar in it's simplest form. e.g glucose.

Micro is interpreted as small size. For example, microcephally is small size of head that is not normal.

Tomy is interpreted as when incision is made into an organ surgically. For example, colonotomy is surgical incision into the colon.

Metry is interpreted as measurement. For example, optometry is (opto+metry). This is (eye+measurement). Which is eye measurement.

Meso is interpreted as middle. For example, mesoderm is the middle layer of the germ layer.

Mening is interpreted as meninges. For example, meningitis is (mening+itis). This is (meninges+inflammation). Which is inflammation of the meninges.

Meno is interpreted as menstruation. For example, menopause is (meno+pause). This is (menstruation+stop). Which is stop of menstruation.

Melan is interpreted as melanin.

Thermo is interpreted as temperature. For example, thermometer is (thermo+meter). This is (temperature+measuring instrument). Which is measuring

instrument of temperature.

Megaly is interpreted as

enlargement that is not normal. For

example, splenomegaly is

(spleno+megaly). This is

(spleen+enlargement that is not

normal). Which is spleen

enlargement that is not normal.

Mal is interpreted as abnormality.

For example, malnutrition is

(mal+nutrition). This is

(abnormality+nutrition). Which is abnormality in nutrition.

Macro is interpreted as large size. For example, macrocephaly is large size head that is not normal.

Ology is interpreted as study of. For example, Ophthalmology is the study of the eye.

Lith is interpreted as stone. For example, nephrolith is (nephro+lith). This is (kidney+stone). Which is kidney stone.

Lipo is interpreted as lipid. For example, lipodosis is lipid metabolism disorder.

Leuco is interpreted as white. For example, leucocyte is (leuco+cyte). This is (white+cell). Which is white blood cell.

Laryngo is interpreted as larynx. For example, laryngotomy is (laryngo+tomy). This is (larynx+surgical incision). Which is surgical incision into the larynx.

Laparo is interpreted as abdomen. For example, laparoscopy is used to perform surgical operation in the abdomen.

Lalia is interpreted as speech. For example, bradylalia is (Brady+lalia). This is (slow+speech). Which is slow speech.

Lact is interpreted as milk. For example, lactation is breast production of milk.

Labio is interpreted as lips. For example, labiopathy is (labio+pathy).

This is (lips+disease). Which is disease of the lips.

Kypho is interpreted as hump. For example, the back kyphosis.

Karyo is interpreted as cell nucleus. For example, karyoblast is cell nucleus formation.

Jejun is interpreted as jejunum. For example, jejunitis is (jejun+itis). This is (jejunum+inflammation). Which is inflammation of the jejunum.

Itis is interpreted as inflammation. For example, arthritis is (arthr+itis).

This is (joint+inflammation). Which is joint inflammation.

Hystero is interpreted as uterus. For example, hysterorrhaphy is (hystero+rrhaphy). This is (uterus+surgical suturing repair). Which is surgical suturing repair of torn uterus.

Hypo is interpreted as low. For example, hypotension is low blood pressure.

Hypno is interpreted as sleep. For example, hypnotics are drugs that make somebody sleep.

Hex is interpreted as six. For example, hexose is sugar having six carbon.

Hernio is interpreted as hernia. For example, herniorrhaphy is (hernio+rrhaphy). This is (hernia +surgical suturing repair). Which is surgical suturing repair of hernia.

Heredo is interpreted as heredity. For example, heredopathy is (heredo+pathy). This is

(heredity+disease). Which is

heredity of disease from parent to

offspring.

Hepat is interpreted as liver. For

example, hepatitis is (hepat+itis).

This is (liver+inflammation).

Hemi is half. For example,

hemiplegia is (hemi+plegia). This is

(half+paralysis). Which is paralysis of

half part of the body.

Helco is ulcer. For example,

helcocolon is (helco+colon). This is

(ulcer+colon). Which is ulcer of the colon.

Haemo is interpreted as blood. For example, Haemopoiesis is (haemo+poiesis). This is (blood+formation). Which is blood formation.

www.ingramcontent.com/pod-product-compliance
Lightning Source LLC
Chambersburg PA
CBHW021438210526
45463CB00002B/556